Essential Oils Safe for Cats

Essential Oil Recipes Safe for
Cats
for Diffusers, Roller Bottles,
Inhalers & more.

Rica V. Gadi

This book is dedicated to all the strong people who are taking responsibility for your own well being and doing something to be better.

All my heartfelt gratitude to the following people: my mom Ruby Jane, you have made me everything I am today; my dad Nestor-- my eternal, my angel, and the source of my perseverance; Mommyling, my spiritual guide ; Ria & Joe, the true witnesses of my transformation and my foundation pillars; Ellie Jane, the sparkle of our eyes;

Juan, thanks for always encouraging me to push harder - you are my ONE; Rocco & Radha, my reason for everything.

The Love of my family and friends is the fountain of inspiration that never runs dry. Thank you for constantly inspiring me, motivating me, and loving me unconditionally.

This book will never be complete without the help of my trusted and talented friends the #NOWsuperstars and my #oilbularya friends

Blending Essential Oils to use for a very specific reason has become very popular in recent years. There are several reasons why this is so. Blending EOs is basically about inhaling - as it has been proven that aromas have the ability to trigger feelings, emotions and personal memories.

With this in mind, it is obvious that everyone is unique when it comes to what triggers your senses. It all boils down to personal preference for the aroma to trigger what you want to unleash. Everyone is different and we all connect to the aroma differently, so what might work for one might not work for another person.

Of course, we also want the blend we personalize to be therapeutic. This is the best reason why to blend essential oils. We want the blend we create to help us with a very specific emotion or physical conditions. As much as smelling good is important in a blend, it is more important that we blend oils that are not only pleasing to the smell but also produces the therapeutic effect we are after.

Then you have to think about contraindications. Making sure the blend you create is safe to use.

I suggest that before blending, find out if the oils you are using are safe for a condition you may have, for example, if you are pregnant, or have specific allergies. Consult your physician prior to moving forward.

The recipes I have in this book is a compilation of what has proven to work and favored by hundreds of EO enthusiasts. It takes out the guesswork to get you started.

Again, we urge you to read the recipes and make sure that this is safe for you to try.

The book is very specific to a physical and emotional condition. There are several recipes here because you might want to rotate and you may like one and not the other. There are also a variety of applications. Some of us prefer to diffuse, some to make roller bottles, and others to create inhalers and sprays.

I hope you enjoy this compilation, feel free to use the notes section and jot down your fave blends. There is a wonderful world of EO blending - this is just the beginning.

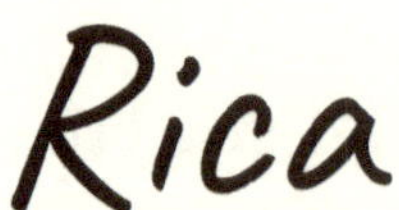

Similar to humans, pets come in all shapes and sizes. Cats have different types, which means that they have different genetic traits in their body. Taking care of cats can be challenging and it is important to know their needs and to monitor their body. As pet owners, we will find all ways to help them grow and be healthy. There are several health fads going around online and one of them is the use of essential oils in aromatherapy. It is evident that this form of alternative treatment is compatible and effective for humans, but the question is, can these oils also be used to benefit cats?

Cats have very strong senses and are very susceptible to odor particles. This is the first thing to observe when deciding to use essential oils for cats. Essential oils are high concentrations of plant extracts that need to be diluted before use, even for humans. Its potency can be something that can cause irritation in cats if not properly handled. On the bright side, their high concentrations mean that they pack a lot of beneficial properties for the body. In most cases when essential oils are used for cats, it is diluted in water first in an 80% to 90% ratio. Some essential oils can be bought in hydrosol form, which is a safer variant for cats as they are already mixed with water. Essential oils must be used with care and with proper instructions from veterinarians.

There are simple rules to follow in order to successfully use essential oils on cats. First of all, the owners must make sure that the essential oils used are 100,% pure and of high quality because there are essential oils in the market that claim to be pure but have already been mixed with other foreign ingredients. Once you have done your research and gathered essential oils that are safe for your cat, testing their compatibility with it would be the next step. You may dab a few essential oils on a tissue and bring it around you to make your cat acclimate to the scent or to observe if they are having reactions to it. It is important to have a place where your cat can stay away from the smell if ever it leads to irritation. It is also not recommended to apply essential oils topically or be ingested but there are some that can be mixed with flea medicine to improve its effectiveness. In these situations, it is crucial to avoid application to your cat's ears and eyes. For any sign of discomfort, seek the help of your doctor.

Essential oils that should never go near your cats are those that are rich in phenol and have citrusy properties.

Table of Contents

Essential Oils Safe for Cats

The Blending Process

These EOs are categorized by aromas, and EOs from the same group usually blend fantastically together.

- Floral – Lavender, Geranium, Jasmine
- Woodsy – Pine, Cedarwood
- Earthy – Vetiver, Patchouli
- Herbaceous – Marjoram, Rosemary, Basil
- Minty – Peppermint, Spearmint, Wintergreen
- Medicinal – Eucalyptus, Frankincense, Melaleuca
- Spicy – Pepper, Clove, Cinnamon
- Oriental – Ginger, Patchouli
- Citrus – Wild Orange, Lemon, Lime

Select oils that will give you the health benefits you are looking to remedy. For increased energy choose: Grapefruit, Lemon, Orange, or Citrus. For Calming and Relaxation choose: Lavender, Cedarwood, or Chamomile. You are encouraged to experiment and play with your oils to see which blends work for you.

TIPS:

- Combine Floral EOs with Woodsy, Spicy and Citrus aromas
- Minty EOs with Woodsy, Earthy, Herbaceous and Citrus aromas
- Earthy EOs with Woodsy and Minty aromas
- Citrus EOs with Floral, Woodsy, Minty, Spicy and Oriental aromas

Essential Oils Substitution List

Sometimes we want to blend oils but we just don't have all the oils as stated in a recipe. I've created an easy to use guide for substitution.

Name of Oil	SUB 1	SUB 2	SUB 3
Arborvitae	Melissa	Cedarwood	Patchouli
Basil	Massage Blend	Marjoram	Thyme
Bergamot	Grapefruit	Lime	
Birch	Wintergreen	Cypress	
Black Pepper	Copaiba	Juniper Berry	Clove
Blue Tansy	Roman Chamomile		
Cardamom	Lavender	Clary Sage	Roman Chamomile
Cassia	Cinnamon		
Cedarwood	Arborvitae	Patchouli	Vetiver
Cellular Blend	Frankincense	Thyme	Clove
Cilantro	Coriander	Cardamom	Black Pepper
Cinnamon	Cassia		
Clary Sage	Ylang Ylang		
Clove	Cassia	Cinnamon	
Copaiba	Thyme	Oregano	Clove
Coriander	Lavender	Juniper Berry	Cardamom

Cypress	Douglas Fir	Massage Blend	Copaiba
Detoxification Blend	Geranium	Copaiba	Rosemary
Digestive Blend	Fennel	Peppermint	Ginger
Dill	Bergamot	Lemon	Wild Orange
Douglas Fir	Siberian Fir	Cypress	
Eucalyptus	Respiratory Blend	Melaleuca	Melissa
Frankincense	Cedarwood		
Geranium	Copaiba	Rose	
Ginger	Digestive Blend	Fennel	Geranium
Grapefruit	Bergamot	Lemon	Wild Orange
Helichrysum	Myrrh		
Jasmine	Roman Chamomile	Rose	Ylang Ylang
Juniper Berry	Coriander		
Lavender	Petitgrain	Roman Chamomile	Coriander
Lemon	Wild Orange	Lime	Grapefruit
Lemongrass	Helichrysum	Cilantro	
Marjoram	Basil	Cypress	
Melaleuca	Neroli	Rosemary	Eucalyptus
Melissa	Black Pepper	Eucalyptus	

Metabolic Blend	Ginger	Peppermint	Cinnamon
Myrrh	Sandalwood	Spikenard	
Neroli	Rosemary	Melissa	Melaleuca
Oregano	Thyme	Basil	Copaiba
Patchouli	Vetiver	Focus Blend	Cedarwood
Peppermint	Spearmint		
Petitgrain	Lavender	Wild Orange	Bergamot
Protective Blend	Cinnamon	Clove	Copaiba
Renewing Blend	Bergamot	Juniper Berry	Myrrh
Respiratory Blend	Eucalyptus	Rosemary	Melaleuca
Roman Chamomile	Blue Tansy	Lavender	Focus Blend
Rose	Geranium	Jasmine	Ylang Ylang
Rosemary	Melaleuca	Neroli	Eucalyptus
SandalWood	Cedarwood	Spikenard	Myrrh
Siberian Fir	Douglas Fir	White Fir	Cedarwood
Soothing Blend	Helichrysum	Peppermint	Wintergreen
Spearmint	Peppermint	Reassuring Blend	
Spikenard	Myrrh	Vetiver	Patchouli
Thyme	Oregano	Copaiba	Clove

Vetiver	Patchouli	Spikenard	Cedarwood
White Fir	Siberian Fir	Douglas Fir	
Wild Orange	Tangerine	Lemon	Grapefruit
Wintergreen	Birch	Siberian Fir	
Ylang Ylang	Jasmine	Lavender	

Diffuse

Diffusing Essential Oils is the safest method to enjoy Essential Oils without the risk of an allergic reaction.

Diffusing Essential Oils
Some Tidbits You Need To Know

Our sense of smell is one of our most powerful senses, and as you have noticed in your own experience, some scents affect you more positively in your minds than others. The body contains over 1,000 receptors for smell—way more receptors than for any of our other senses.

Diffusion Essential Oils means the process vaporizes oils into the air by releasing tiny amounts into the air. Inhalation is totally safe and is super low risk. Chances of any EO rising to dangerous levels while diffusion is slim to none.

Diffusing Essential Oils around newborns, babies, young children, pregnant or nursing women, and pets should be done with caution. Read up on safety.

It is advisable that Diffusing Essential Oils for only about 15-30 minutes at a time to be most effective. NEVER leave your diffuser on overnight. Make sure your diffuser is filled with the right amount of water and you understand the operating directions.

While diffusing essential oils, be sure that your space has great ventilation. Crack a window open if the scent becomes strong.

Never add Carrier Oils to your diffuser. This may cause your diffuser to malfunction. Clean your diffuser at least 3 times a week with warm water and natural soap to ensure the diffuser is well maintained and bacteria and mold does not accumulate.

Diffusing Essential Oils
Basic Guidelines

Just a few things you need to know and prepare before getting started Diffusing Essential Oils.

Things you need:
Ultrasonic Oil Diffuser
Essential Oils
Water

Just follow the number of drops in the recipe, drop on to an oil diffuser and fill the rest with water.

All diffusers are different and will have its own water minimum and maximum level. Read the diffuser instruction before use.

Ideally, it is best to diffuse for 15-30 minutes and turn off the diffuser. The effect should be good for at least 2-3 hours. Turn your diffuser back on after 3 hours to reinforce oil diffusing effects.

It is not advisable to use EO in humidifiers.

These are not made to release EOS

Roll

Essential Oil Roller Bottles is the easiest method to enjoy Essential Oils Anywhere and Whenever.

Essential Oils are usually super concentrated and too hard to measure how much to actually put straight from the bottle.

Roller bottles are a way that you are able to create blends ready to use with the right dilution. It allows your EO to last longer.

It also makes it easier to apply exactly where you want to target without getting it all over the place.

It is handy and easy to carry in your purse, ready to use at any time you want to.

I like to apply EOs at the bottom of the feet for many reasons. Our feet have bigger pores than any other skin in our bodies. This means that they are able to suck in the therapeutic compounds in our blend into the bloodstream faster than any other parts of the body. Imagine comparing a normal straw to an oversized straw and how much more you can suck in with the latter. This is how the soles of our feet are compared to the rest of the skin in our bodies.

The skin on our feet is also less sensitive and is designed to withstand some abuse. The risk of having an irritation from EOS is less likely to happen when applied on the feet.

The feet don't have the glands that act as a barrier. Sebaceous glands are glands in our skin that produce an oily substance called Sebum, for the purpose of lubricating and waterproofing the skin. Since this is oil and if you put oil on top of oil, it can act as a barrier or it may slow down penetration.

The feet and palms of our hands are the only skin that don't have these, so it is ideal to apply Essential Oils to the feet for maximum penetration.

Now, it would be hard to apply oils directly and very messy, right? Roller bottles make it super easy and convenient to roll the EOs at the bottom of our feet.

Carrier Oils Info

Carrier oils are vegetable-based oils with their own healing properties that dilute essential oils used to help carry the EOs into the skin.

Essential oils are highly concentrated and could evaporate very quickly. The carrier oil is mixed with the essential oil so it could penetrate the skin before it actually evaporates. Although EOs are oils, it is actually not that oily. When mixed with a carrier oil, it allows you to have more of the essential oil into your skin without wasting EOS to evaporate, making the healing properties of the EO strong and more effective.

There are also Essential oils that are too strong to apply directly to the skin and may cause damage, so it is important to dilute them with carrier oil.

Never add Carrier Oils to your diffuser. This may cause your diffuser to malfunction. Clean your diffuser at least 3 times a week with warm water and natural soap to ensure the diffuser is well maintained and bacteria and mold does not accumulate.

Carrier Oils

There are a lot of different carrier oils that you can use with EOs to dilute them in a roller bottle.

To name a few :

Almond Oil - moisturizing and stays liquid at room temperature. Do not use it if you are allergic to nuts.

Apricot Kernel Oil - moisturizing and suitable for sensitive skin or kids. It is super gentle on the skin.

Avocado Oil - moisturizing and suitable for sensitive and damaged skin. Perfect for skin problems.Can be mixed with other carrier oils

Castor Oil - with antibacterial, antiviral and antifungal properties, use topically to eliminate pain and relieve skin irritation.

Coconut Oil - its antibacterial, antiviral and antifungal properties it is the best and most versatile for skin care. The skin absorbs this very quickly. It solidifies in room temp and may still have a slight coconut oil aroma in it - but you can get fractionated coconut oil to eliminate the 2 challenges above.

Grapeseed Oil - not just for cooking but also great for topical application on the skin.

Jojoba Oil - one of my faves for skin care blends. This oil is the closest to our natural oil our skin produces so it is absorbed easily without being oily. Also amazing for massage oil blends.

Olive Oil - this is the oil for herb type oils. mostly used for cooking but can also be applied to the skin but would need to be blended with a carrier oil that is mild and absorb well with the skin.

Rosehip Seed Oil - super good for deep moisturizing or skin irritations. This oil has a high content of antioxidants and helps remedy dry, scarred and wounded skin.

Recommended Roller Bottle Dilution Guide

RECOMMENDED ROLL-ON BOTTLE DILUTION AMOUNTS

5 ml (1/6 oz.) Roll-on Bottle = ~100 drops (1tsp.)
10 ml (1/3 oz.) Roll-on Bottle = ~200 drops (2 tsp.)
30 ml. (1 oz.) Roll-on Bottle = ~600 drops (6 tsp.)

Roll-on Size	5 ml	10 ml	30 ml	Add EO drops to roll-on, then fill with carrier oil.	
Essential Oil Drops	1	2	6	1%	Dilution Percentage
	2	4	12	2%	
	3	6	18	3%	
	5	10	30	5%	
	10	20	60	10%	
	20	40	120	20%	
	25	50	150	25%	
	50	100	300	50%	

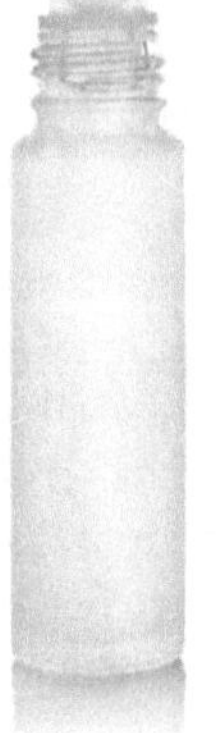
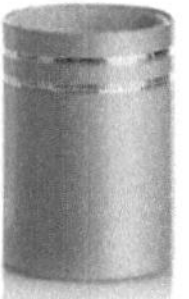

General Guidelines:
Birth to 12 months = .3-.5% dilution
1-5 years = 1.5-3% dilution
6-11 years = 1.5-5% dilution
12-17 years = 1.5-20% dilution
18 years and older = 1.5% dilution-Neat (no dilution)
Elderly or Sensitive Skin = 1-3% dilution
Daily Use = 2-5% dilution
Short Term Use = 10-25% dilution
Local Skin or Systemic Issues = 50% dilution-Neat

These are general guidelines suggestions--not absolute rules--based on traditional aromatheraphy practice.
(Kurt Schnaubelt PhD, Valerie Worwood, Robert Tisserand)

Dilution Basics:

How much you dilute your EO depends on different factors such as weight, sensitivity, health conditions, EOs that are blended in or how long that blend has been used for. There is never an absolute dilution rule, it is you who knows about your level and tolerance. I feel that it is best to start with a higher dilution percentage and increase EO drops over time.

To make sure your EO is safe, make sure that the oils you use are therapeutic grade and do your research on the source and extraction methods used to produce the oils.

Roller Bottle Blending Order

I normally just start with dropping the drops of oil into the **10mL roller bottle**, then adding the carrier oil up until the shoulder of the bottle. Capping the bottle off with the roller and the bottle cap. Instead of shaking the bottle, I like to roll the bottle between my palms first for a minute or 2 for blending, then finishing it off with a few shakes.

NOTE: All recipes in this book are for a 10mL Roller Bottle. If you have a bigger or smaller roller bottle, adjust the number of EO drops based on the size of your bottle.

Inhale

Essential Oil Inhalers are the most convenient way to enjoy Essential Oils Anywhere and Whenever.

Essential Oil Inhalers give you quick and easy access to the vast therapeutic benefits of essential oils.

Blending Essential Oils in an Inhaler Some Tidbits You Need To Know

EO Inhalers or aroma sticks are compact tubes, with a cotton wick inside and a protective cover, to lock the aroma within.

Your preferred blend of essential oils is absorbed by the cotton wick, and safely enclosed in a tube that fits inside of the cover. The cover is easily removed for access to the tube to breathe in the aroma. Usually lasts about 3 months, depending on the oil blend used.

I absolutely love these because they encourage me to take a moment during super stressful moments, and just breathe.

It is in times of stress when our breathing patterns often change and taking deep breaths promote a feeling of calm and inner peace. Breath work combined with visualization plus a relaxing inhaler, can offer relief to symptoms of stress and help your body to come back to the state of homeostasis.

Aroma Sticks can be carried in your tiny purse, even compact enough to fit in your pocket. You can enjoy your favorite EOs anywhere and you can use them with discretion.

I love diffusing, and do all the time but not everyone in my space may enjoy the scents I enjoy or they may not benefit from the therapeutic benefits of the EOs I am diffusing - so the inhaler is one way to not only enjoy my choice of blends but to keep in personal not affecting everyone else around me.

Inhalers not only benefits me but also keep those around me safe in case the oils I want to blend may pose a risk to those around me who may have a health issue not advised to be exposed to my choice EOs/

When making Aroma Sticks, You may use your chosen EOs at 100% Concentration.

Inhaler Basic Guidelines

Breathe in slow and deep to absorb the EO molecules directly into your olfactory system.

Inhalers are super easy to use. You just remove the cap and inhale from the inhaler tube, count 1 to 5 slowly as you inhale. The EO molecules get drawn into our bloodstream through our nasal cavity and get delivered throughout our entire body.

Simple to use, easy to carry, portable and compact. You never have to be without your favorite blends, ever.

Inhaler Blending Basics

Inhalers are super easy and simple to make.

All you need is an inhaler set which consist of the following:

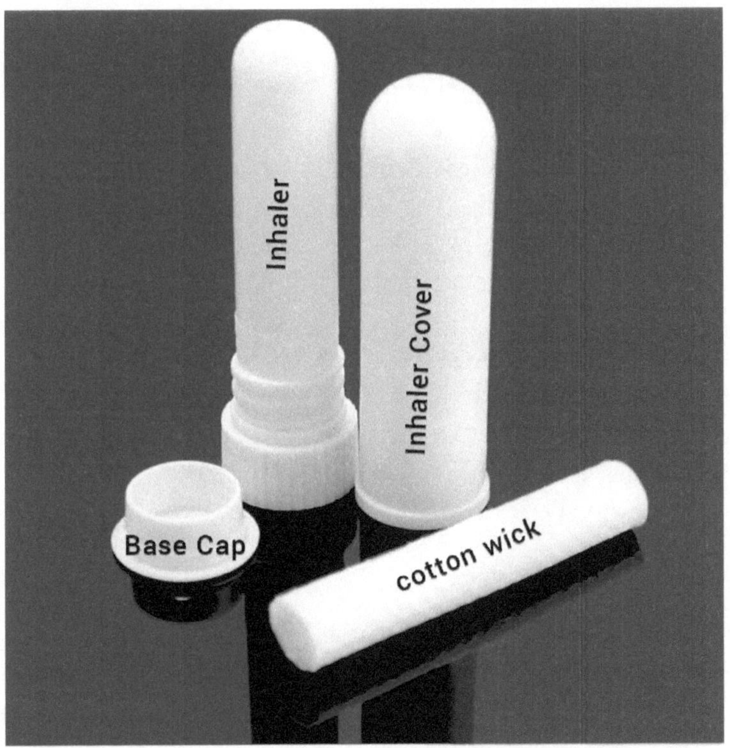

Inhaler, Inhaler Cover, Base Cap and Cotton Wick.

You will need your Essential Oils.

I like to use a pipette for precision and a small petri dish so I can see the oil.

Blending is super easy, just combine the drops and swirl it around in the petri dish and when you are satisfied you can go ahead and drop the cotton wick to absorb all the oil in the dish.

Once the wick is ready you can drop it in the inhaler and cap the bottom with the Base Cap. I usually like to secure the cover with the inhaler so I don't have to do it later.

I usually use 15-20 drops of EO total in a recipe and it can last up to 3 months. Some recipes will need more but on average it is in this range.

EO Recipes Safe for Cats

Homemade Spray

30 drops Geranium
30 drops Citronella
20 drops Lemon
20 drops Lavender
10 drops Rosemary
1 tbsp Vodka or Rubbing Alcohol
½ cup Natural Witch Hazel
½ cup Water (or vinegar)
1 tbsp Vegetable Glycerin (optional)

Put the essential oils in a glass splash bottle. Include alcohol or vodka and shake well to mix it together.
Put in witch hazel and shake to join.
Include ½ tsp vegetable glycerin if utilizing. This isn't important yet helps everything remain joined.
Include water and shake once more, shake before each utilization as the oils and water will normally isolate some after some time.

Nourishing Neroli Vitamin E Cream

2 oz Softened Shea Butter
444 drops Vitamin E Oil
7 drops Pure Neroli Essential Oil
1/2 tbsp Raw honey (optional)

Into a Magic Bullet, include 2 oz of relaxed
shea spread, 1/2 tsp nutrient E oil and 7
drops of unadulterated neroli basic oil.
For more skin feeding impacts, include 1/2
tsp of crude nectar.
Mix for a couple of moments till smooth.
Move into a 4 oz golden glass container.
Apply a pea-sized measure of this cream all
over your face, or just on the skin break out
scars each prior night bed.
You can likewise apply this under cosmetics
in the first part of the day.

DIY Moisturizing Fleas Block Bar

1 oz Coconut Oil (organic, unrefined)
1 oz Beeswax (organic)
1 oz Shea Butter (organic)
10 drops Geranium
10 drops Citronella
Double boiler

Metal utensil (I use a spoon)
Molds, paper lined muffin cups or twist up tubes.
Put the essential oils in a glass splash bottle.
Include alcohol or vodka and shake well to mix it.
Put in witch hazel and shake to join.
Include ½ tsp vegetable glycerin if utilizing. This isn't important yet helps everything remain joined.
Include water and shake once more, shake before each utilization as the oils and water will normally isolate some after some time.

Roman Chamomile Cream

1 drop Roman Chamomile

Roman chamomile helps balance and calms.
It also aids wound healing by reducing inflammation and relieving pain.
Use in spray or palm method.

Frankincense Cream

1 drop Frankincense

Frankincense aids the healing of injuries, itching, allergies and infections.
Use 1 drop as a swab or try it on your cat's collar or apply the palm method.

Rosemary Spray

1 drop Rosemary Essential Oil

Rosemary will calm and settle your cat.
Use 1 drop in a spray bottle or use a palm
method.
Place a few drops on your collar, blanket or
favourite toy.
Use as a swab for minor injuries.
Make sure to source a top quality Lavandula
angustifolia and not an inferior
camphor-rich rosemary for use on cats.

Rosemary Spray

1-2 drops Rosemary
Water

Rosemary baths can be wonderful for flea
control.
Most prefer to mix one or two drops into a
pitcher of water and pour the mixture over
your cat and let it dry without rinsing.
However, if your cat isn't fond of water or
you just want to be on the safe side, consider
using it alongside the cedar wood oil on
your cat's collar and in the spray.

Lemongrass Spray

Water
2-3 drops Lemongrass Oil

Much like with cedar wood, lemongrass essential oil is great for keeping fleas and other pests at bay without harming your feline friend.
Try to fill up a glass spray bottle with water and mix in two to three drops of peppermint oil.
Don't spray it directly on your cat, but rather around the furniture, bedding, and carpet. However, you can dip a flea comb into the diluted mixture and then comb it through your cat's fur.

Cedarwood Spray

1-2 drops Cedarwood Oil
Vinegar/Alcohol
Water
10 drops Cedarwood Oil

Not only is cedarwood safe for cats, but it actually has been proven to be lethal to adult fleas.
After you have given your cat a flea bath, try adding a drop or two of cedar wood oil into their collar in order to prevent future flea infestations.
Additionally, you can use cedar wood in a spray for fabrics in order to kill the fleas as their hatching.
We would recommend a spray with equal parts vinegar or alcohol and water in a glass spray bottle with around 10 drops of cedar wood oil per cup of liquid.

Flea and Tick Spray

1 16oz Spray Bottle
Spring Water
8 drops Sweet Orange
8 drops Lavender
8 drops Lemongrass
12 drops Geranium
20 drops Patchouli
20 drops Cedarwood Atlas

Start by mixing every essential oil to the 16oz splash bottle.
After that, put it to your shoulder with water (not water from the tap)
Mix for a long time before use.

Flea & Tick Repellent Spray

5 drops of Lavender
2 drops Citronella
2 drops of Cedarwood
2 drops of Lemongrass
2 tbsp of Carrier oil
12-16 oz Spray Bottle (use a 16-ounce bottle if this mixture is too strong)

Mix all the ingredients to your splash bottle and fill with water.

Flea-Be-Gone Shampoo

1 cup Water (distilled is best, but tap water is fine, too)
2/3 cup Castile Soap
197 drops Olive Oil
20-30 drops Essential Oil (Lavender or Peppermint)

Put the essential oils in a glass splash bottle. Include alcohol or vodka and shake well to mix it.
Put in witch hazel and shake to join.
Include ½ tsp vegetable glycerin if utilizing.
This isn't important yet helps everything remain joined.
Include water and shake once more.
Shake before each utilization as the oils and water will normally isolate some after some time.

Flea-Free Spritz

1 tsp Vegetable Glycerin
½ oz (15 ml) Grain Alcohol (Vodka)
98 drops Sulfated Castor Oil
7 oz Distilled or Spring Water
10 drops Grapefruit Seed Extract (not essential oil)
4 drops Clary Sage
1 drop Citronella
7 drops Peppermint
3 drops Lemon

Blend all the ingredients into a bottle.
Store in a dark or opaque glass or plastic spritz bottle.
Shake well before use.

"Shoo, Flea, Don't Bother Me" Powder

1 cup food-grade Diatomaceous Earth
½ cup Bentonite Clay Powder
¼ cup Rosemary Leaf Powder
¼ cup Black Walnut Hull Powder
5 drops Cedarwood
5 drops Rosemary

Mix the DE or potentially BC with other dry ingredients indicated in a medium bowl and tenderly speed to mix.
Include the essential oils, spreading the drops around the powder, and whisk again to mix.
Freely spoon the blend into the compartment, at that point shake energetically for around 30 seconds.
Mark and date the powder. Enable the powder to synergism for 24 hours before use.
Store at room temperature, away from warmth and light; use inside 1 year.

Bite Ban Flea & Tick Powder

1½ cups Food-Grade Diatomaceous Earth
¼ cup Lemongrass Powder
¼ cup Neem Leaf Powder
10 drops Lemongrass Essential Oil

Mix the DE or potentially BC with other dry ingredients indicated in a medium bowl and tenderly speed to mix.
Include the essential oils, spreading the drops around the powder, and whisk again to mix.
Freely spoon the blend into the compartment, at that point shake energetically for around 30 seconds.
Mark and date the powder.
Enable the powder to synergism for 24 hours before use.
Store at room temperature, away from warmth and light; use inside 1 year.

Apple Cider Vinegar Flea Shampoo

1 cup of Apple Cider Vinegar
1 quart of Warm Water
1 cup of Liquid Dish Soap

First, you should mix the warm water and
apple cider vinegar together in a large bowl.
Once these two ingredients are combined,
slowly add the liquid dish soap.
Mix all of these ingredients together, then
pour them into a spray bottle.
Once it is in the bottle, give it a gentle shake
to ensure everything is properly combined.

Eucalyptus Cats Shampoo

7 drops Eucalyptus Oil

Blending 7 drops of Eucalyptus oil to a 32-oz.
a cleanser jug would make this
arrangement a convincing specialist for the
insects to relinquish your pet's body.

Lemon Flea Shampoo

1/2 cup of Fresh Squeezed Lemon Juice
1 1/2 to 2 cups of Warm Water
1/4 to 1/2 cup of Baby Shampoo or Castile
Soap

The first step is to squeeze 1/2 of a cup
of lemon juice and add it to a
medium-sized bowl.
Once this is done, add your warm water to
the lemon
juice and mix it well.
Finally, add your baby shampoo or castile
soap to the
lemon juice and water.
Stir until everything is incorporated, and
store it in a glass jar or container until you're
ready to use it.

Natural Dry Flea Shampoo

1 cup Baking Soda
1 cup Cornstarch
2 to 4 drops of Lavender or Lemon Essential
Oil

Start by putting the baking soda and
cornstarch in a medium bowl.
Mix
them together until they're combined.
Next, add the essential oil to the mix.
Start with two drops of the essential oil of
your choosing and add more if you
have to.

Your Own EO Blends

<u>Book Ordering</u>

To order your copy / copies of

*Essential Oils
Safe for Cats*

please visit: **EOrecipes.net**

You can also check out other titles
available.

Bulk Pricing and
Affiliate Programs Available